Contents

1

THE
PUBLIC FACE
OF THE
Geisha
—— 4 ——

2

THE
PRIVATE FACE
OF THE
Geisha
—— 20 ——

ACKNOWLEDGMENTS

The text for Part One was written by Cecilia Walters.

The text extracts in Part Two were translated by Rachel Kess, and the poems selected from *Eastern Love*, translated by E. Powys Mathers.

The illustration on page 17 is based on an original from *Japanese Music and Musical Instruments* by William P. Malm, published by Charles E. Tuttle, Rutland, Vermont, 1959.

Texts consulted for reference were *Geisha* by Liza Crihfield Dalby, published by University of California Press, Berkeley, California, 1983, *Mysterious Japan* by Julian Street, published by Heinemann, London, 1922, and *Geisha* by Kyoko Aihara, published by Carlton Books, London, 2000.

EDDISON·SADD EDITIONS

Editorial Director Ian Jackson
Proof Reader Jane Struthers

Art Director Elaine Partington
Design Blue Banana Associates Ltd
Illustration Kathy Wyatt
Calligraphy Ruth Rowland
Illustration Reference Diana Morris

Production Charles James and Karyn Claridge

Geisha

SECRETS

A PILLOW BOOK
FOR LOVERS

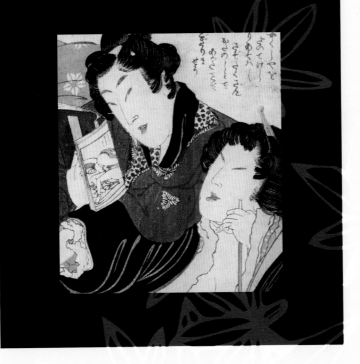

Caroll & Graf Publishers, Inc.
New York

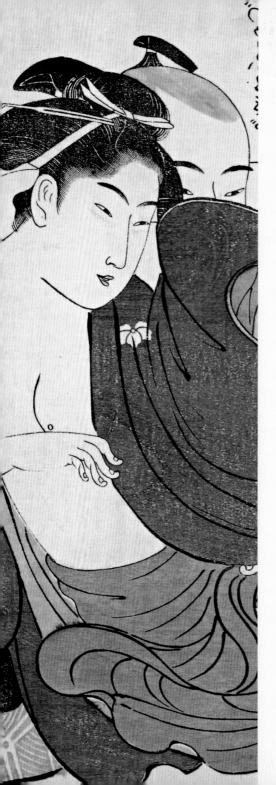

First published in the United States in 2000
By Carroll & Graf Publishers, Inc.

Carroll & Graf Publishers, Inc.
19 West 21st Street
New York, NY 10010
A division of Avalon Publishing Group

ISBN 0-7867-0835-2

Library of Congress Cataloging-in-Publication Data
is available on request

AN EDDISON • SADD EDITION
Edited, designed and produced by
Eddison Sadd Editions Limited
St Chad's House
148 King's Cross Road
London WC1X 9DH

Phototypeset in Gill Sans Light using QuarkXPress on
Apple Macintosh
Origination by Rainbow Graphic Arts, HK
Printed in Hong Kong

Editorial note: Japanese words used only once and immediately followed by a definition have not been included in this glossary.

desho	geisha's most formal kimono
geiko	Kyoto name for a geisha
geta	wooden clogs for bad weather
hanamachi	"flower quarter," a word for a geisha community
karyūkai	"flower and willow world," a poetic term for geisha society
katsura	wig for traditional hairstyles
maiko	Kyoto name for an apprentice geisha
minarai-san	apprentice, literally "learner by observation"
momoware	name for the traditional hairstyle worn by maiko, the "split peach" shimada
obi	wide, heavy sash always worn with a kimono
ochaya	teahouse
ohikizuri	trailing kimono with long sleeves worn by maiko
oiran	courtesan; high-class lady of pleasure in the licensed quarters
okāsan	"mother"; name given to managers of geisha houses and teahouses
okiya	officially recognized lodging house where geisha and maiko live
okobo	high wooden clogs worn by maiko
omisedashi	ceremony celebrating the maiko's debut
onēsan	older sister, in a geisha "family"
sansan-kudo	symbolic exchange of cups of sake; literally, "three times thrice"
shimada	traditional hairstyle worn by geisha
shirabyoshi	dancing girls
shironuri	the white makeup worn by maiko
tabi	white cotton socks worn with kimono
tatami	floor mat made of straw
ukiyo	literally "floating world," the pleasure society of feudal Japan

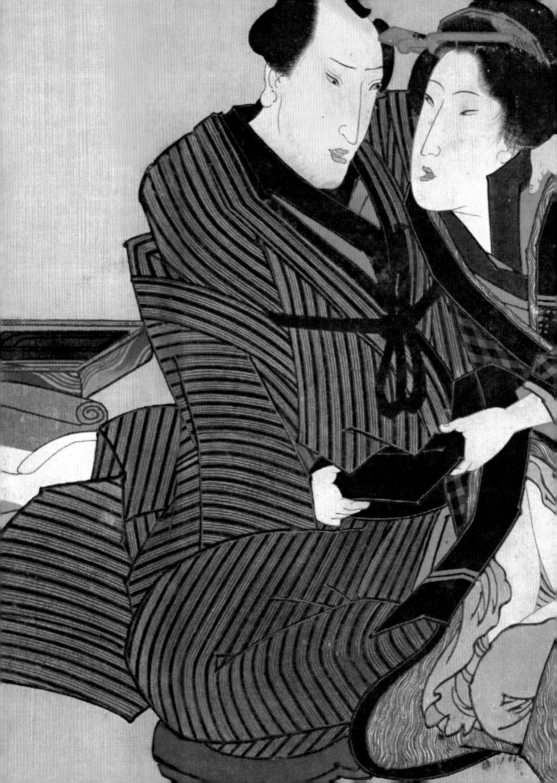

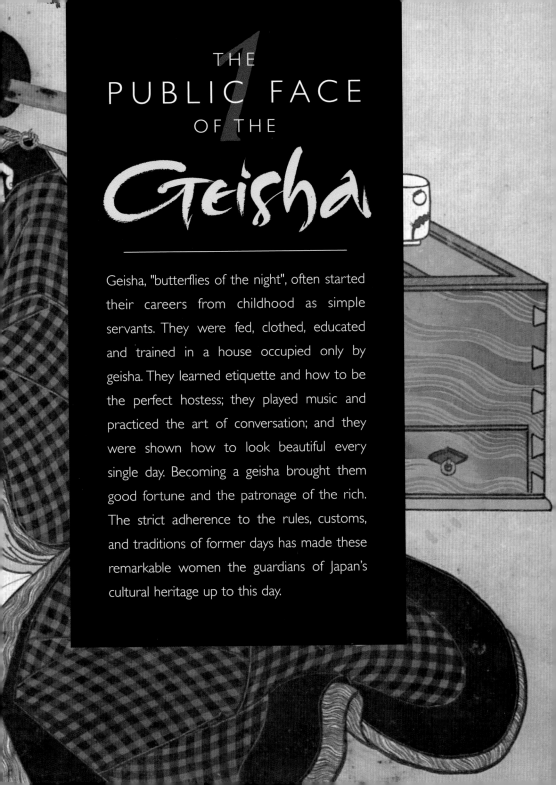

THE PUBLIC FACE OF THE *Geisha*

Geisha, "butterflies of the night", often started their careers from childhood as simple servants. They were fed, clothed, educated and trained in a house occupied only by geisha. They learned etiquette and how to be the perfect hostess; they played music and practiced the art of conversation; and they were shown how to look beautiful every single day. Becoming a geisha brought them good fortune and the patronage of the rich. The strict adherence to the rules, customs, and traditions of former days has made these remarkable women the guardians of Japan's cultural heritage up to this day.

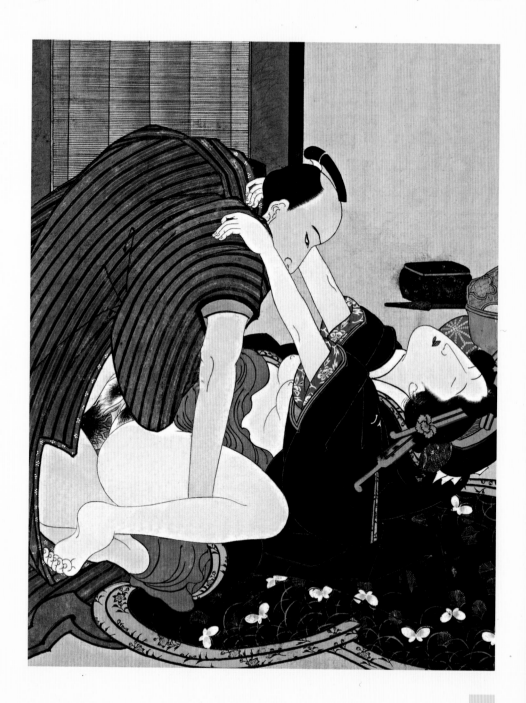

HIS PRETTY GESTURE

Because of his pretty gesture
I have fallen completely in love with him.

My letter written in common character
Will be worth more than a verbal message.
But I may not hold him yet.
I am going to drink sake all night
Without bothering to warm it.

I lie down on the floor
Just where I am, and sleep.
I wake with a start
To hear the night watch crying:
"Fire, take care of fire."

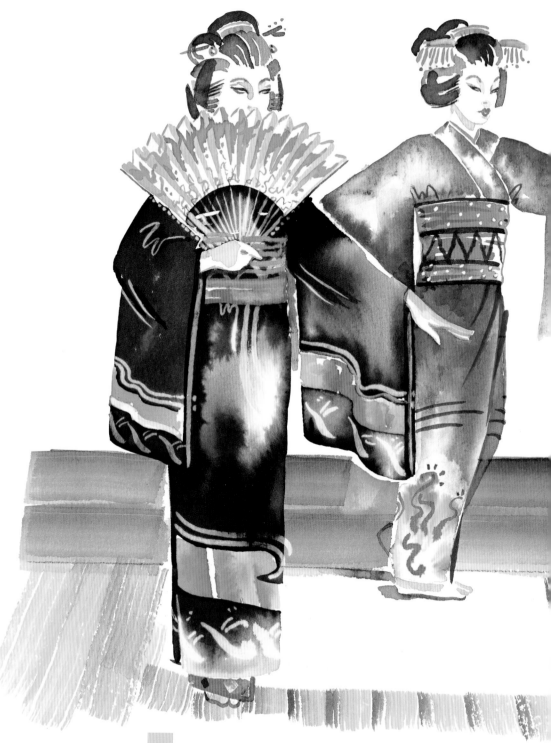

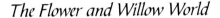

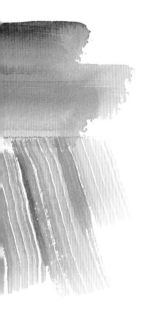

The Flower and Willow World

"Nothing is more silent than the beginning of a Japanese banquet, and no one, except a native, could possibly imagine the tumultuous ending.

"The guests take their places noiselessly; maidens whose bare feet make no sound lay lacquered services upon the matting. All present bow silently, take up their *bashi* (chopsticks), and fall to. But bashi, deftly used, cannot be heard at all. The maidens pour warm sake into the cup of each guest without making the least sound; and it is not until several dishes have been emptied and several cups of sake absorbed, that tongues are loosened.

"Then, all at once, with little bursts of laughter, a number of young girls enter, make the customary prostration of greeting, glide into the open space between the ranks of the guests, and begin to serve the wine with grace and dexterity. They are pretty; they are clad in very costly robes of silk; they are girdled like queens; and the beautifully dressed hair of each is decked with mock flowers, with wonderful combs and pins, and with curious ornaments of gold. They greet the stranger as if they had always known him; they jest, laugh, and utter funny little cries.

"These are the geisha, hired for the banquet. And the banquet, at first so silent, changes to a merry tumult."

Nothing much has changed to this day in the Flower and Willow world, the poetic name for geisha society, since the American writer and journalist, Lafcadio Hearn, wrote these lines in *Glimpses of Unfamiliar Japan* in 1894. Except, of course, the social world around them.

During a banquet, once the sake has been served and guests are relaxed, geisha entertain with dance using traditional accessories—brightly colored fans to exaggerate their hand gestures—and accompanied by the three-stringed shamisen.

7

IN TRADITIONAL JAPAN, *YATSUME-YA*, OR SEX SHOPS, PROVIDED AN
ASTONISHING ARRAY OF MERCHANDISE. IN ADDITION TO EVERY KIND,
SHAPE AND SIZE OF ARTIFICIAL PENIS, THERE WERE ERECTION AIDS,
MASTURBATION DEVICES, CLITORAL STIMULATORS, APHRODISIACS,
LUBRICANTS, CONTRACEPTIVES, BOOKS AND PRINTS FOR INSTRUCTION,
AND THE UBIQUITOUS HYGIENIC TISSUES WITHOUT WHICH JAPANESE
LOVERS WOULD BE LOST. THE AUTHOR OF THIS AMUSING LETTER SEEMS
TO HAVE BEEN A SATISFIED CUSTOMER.

Impossible! I took his *matsuke** in my mouth until my jaw ached, I sucked him until my eyes watered. I chaffed him between my hands. I let him play love's game between my thighs, my buttocks, under my arm, between my breasts. I whispered erotic possibilities in his ear that would tempt a samurai away from boys. But all this was to no avail. He was large—and very red but soft like a lobster claw out of its shell. I warmed a pretty bottle of sake and played on my shamisen until—the servant returned. She smiled knowingly, but mercifully my protector did not see. It was the work of a moment to slip the *namako-no wa** over his disappointment. I loosened my hair and brushed his body with the heavy tresses. My sister, what a transformation! Such a simple remedy and soon my protector and I were joined by a third so imposing that Izanagi and Izanami* could have used it to descend from the sky. The rest, sister, you can imagine!

*Matsuke means mushroom, a popular traditional metaphor in Japan for the penis.

*Otherwise called higo-zuiki, a ring which encourages and maintains erection by temporarily interrupting the return blood supply from the penis.

*In the Shinto creation myth the first male and female slide to earth down a giant phallus.

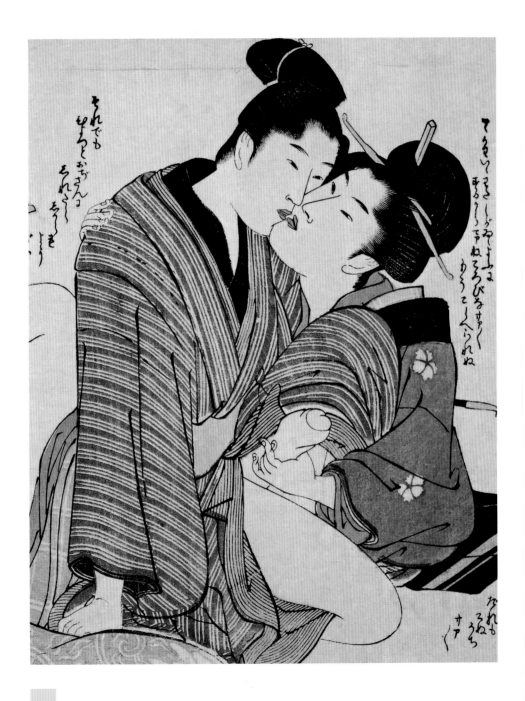

It all began when, in 794, Emperor Kammu, in love with the brilliant culture of Tang China, decided to build a new imperial capital on the same lines as the Chinese capital Changan. Kyoto, first called Heian-kyo, "the peaceful city," became, under the pacific rule of the noble Fujiwara dynasty, the artistic and intellectual capital of Japan.

The most brilliant writer of the period was a woman, Sei Shonagon, author of *Makura-no-soshi*, "The Pillow Book," a journal of erotic thoughts, memories and fantasies which became as famous as its contemporary work, "Tale of Genji," also written by a woman. *Shirabyoshi*, girls who performed dances based on Buddhist prayers, were also mistresses of the warrior class and the nobility.

In 1600, shogun Tokugawa triumphed over his rivals and chose Edo (now Tokyo) to be the seat of his military dictatorship. The rise of the geisha—known as geiko in Kyoto—can be traced to that period.

During the almost three-century long Edo period, the powerful shogun government controlled almost every aspect of life: jobs, travel, food, distribution, and even pleasure. Since many men stayed single their whole lives while fulfilling their duties to their lords, prostitution was seen as a necessary service.

Men who couldn't afford prostitutes had to be satisfied with looking at *shunga* (literally "spring pictures," the same sexual euphemism as *baishun*, or "selling spring," meaning prostitution), the erotic prints that were often published in portfolios of folded pages and which are censored in Japan today.

Prostitution was legal but licensed. Prostitutes were registered as such and geisha had a far more ambiguous relationship with their customers/clients. "The Yoshiwara Pillow"—a sort of sexual guide—was published in 1660, and some of the ladies of the floating world of Edo may have slipped this little book under their pillow expressly for the pleasure of their clients.

Geisha thrived during this period. Originally dancing girls providing musical and visual entertainment at parties, geisha progressed to the stage of pouring sake for guests. In 1712 teahouses were granted licenses so that geisha could entertain there.

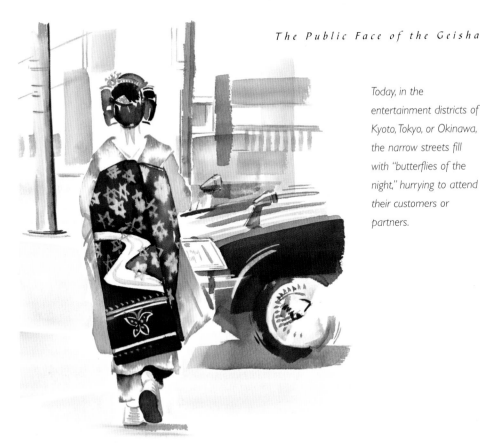

Today, in the entertainment districts of Kyoto, Tokyo, or Okinawa, the narrow streets fill with "butterflies of the night," hurrying to attend their customers or partners.

In the course of the eighteenth century, the term geisha, literally "artist," described various professional women. And men. Geisha in the licensed quarters were forbidden to sleep with the *yujo*'s (courtesans') customers. They were considered to have a social role to play and regarded as a respectable institution.

Geisha were recognized as practicing a distinct profession, and a registry office (*kenban*) was set up to provide and enforce rules of conduct for them. A geisha who openly sold her favors was exposed naked in front of the guild jail. They were not to wear flamboyant kimono, or combs or jeweled pins in their hair, and so on. (Until 1957 the law tried to preserve the distinction.)

In 1870, the new Meiji (meaning "enlightened") emperor moved the imperial capital from Kyoto, and took up residence in Tokyo (Edo). The Meiji period, which lasted until World War I, was one of popularity and

KAWAI, KAWAI
(My dear, my dear)

The firefly singing not
Burns in silence;
She suffers more
Than the loud insect who says:
"Kawai, kawai!"
Why have I given all my soul
To a man without sincerity?
I regret it. I rather regret it.

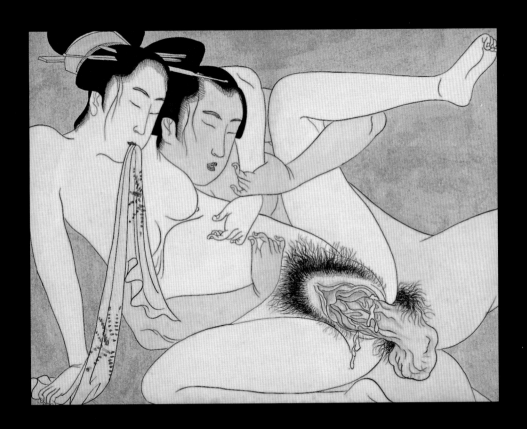

prosperity for the geisha. It is estimated that there were 2,300 geisha in Tokyo in 1905 and, in 1920, the number had grown to 10,000.

Since 1975, geisha have relinquished all claims to being avant-garde, which meant being Westernized. Their image, formed in Japan's feudal past, must be kept, and so today, they look much the same as in 1894. Lafcadio Hearn would recognize them.

Joining the okiya as a young girl, the apprentice geisha has to start at the bottom. She works hard as a maid, taking care of all the household chores, as she undergoes her basic training and classes in song, dance and musicianship.

From Caterpillar to Butterfly

Most geisha begin their careers by actually living in an *okiya*, geisha house, to serve as an "apprentice," *minarai-san*, or *maiko* (exists only in Kyoto). In the past, very young girls were sold to the *hanamachi*, pleasure quarters, by impoverished parents from the countryside to help them feed the rest of their starving families. But today, a girl must stay at school until she is 15 before she can start her apprenticeship in an okiya.

The okiya resembles a family home. It is managed by a "mother," *okasan*, who often is also the owner of an *ochaya*, teahouse, in the hanamachi. The apprentice sleeps and has her meals there, and everything is paid for her—on credit. She will pay back her debts when she has become a successful geiko. She has to go to special school every day, to learn dancing, music and tea ceremony, and follow a very stiff discipline. The okasan is in charge of all matters relating to banquets (*ozashiki*) held in her ochaya, and she will train a minarai-san on how to behave there. But before she becomes even a minarai-san, the apprentice usually acts as a maid, a *shikomi-san*. She must do the house chores, practice her music, and learn her lessons. She has very little free time and life is hard and restricted; she seldom meets boys. Shikomi lasts about a year.

When she becomes a minarai-san, she starts to wear *shironuri*, white paste makeup, and the maiko's *ohikizuri*, a trailing kimono with long full sleeves, and an *obi*, a wide, long sash tied with one end hanging. She will have to learn the difficult deportment involved in wearing this traditional geisha outfit.

The end of this training is followed by *sansan-kudo*, a ceremony that will bond the new maiko with the geiko who will be her *onesan*, older sister, with a triple exchange of sake. The older sister becomes the most important figure in the young maiko's life. It is her responsibility is to teach the maiko all there is to know about life in the hanamachi and also about personal matters.

The rigorous training over, maiko graduates to geiko in an important ceremony. She is helped into a stunning kimono by her dresser and white makeup is applied to her face, neck and shoulders.

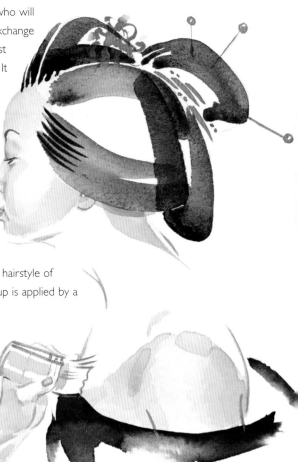

The more important *omisedashi* ceremony follows next day, celebrating the maiko's debut. For this she wears a sumptuous kimono of black crested silk, with a special obi and sash clasp. Her hair is arranged by a hairdresser into the *ware-shinobu*, the first hairstyle of her career as maiko; and her white makeup is applied by a special makeup artist on that day.

The okiya prepares and provides the new maiko's complete wardrobe. It includes kimono for every season, underwear, ornaments, accessories, *tabi* (socks) and *okobo*, high-heeled wooden clogs with bells. The cost is estimated at about 10 million yen (equivalent to over $90,000 today).

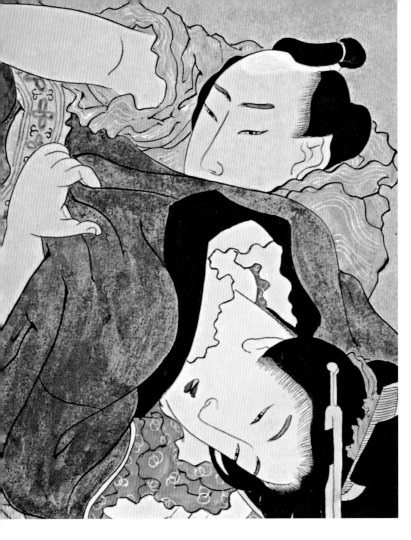

robe and jumped on me. Pushing first the chrysanthemum of my anus
with his pestle, he drops then to the Princess of Flowers and busies
himself there. I am completely filled, and when he pulls back and plunges
in again, I cry out. I cry not with pain but with lust. My lower lips are vocal
too, sucking at this unexpected feast. Riding higher with every thrust, his
loins slap against my buttocks, he the leaping white tiger,* me his prey.
With a lunge and a roar the doctor leaves the royal way. I feel his bonze*
head straining against my chrysanthemum, then the scalding of his fire
juice in my bowels.* As his bell churns, so does mine; my voice answers
his in cries of terrible pleasure.

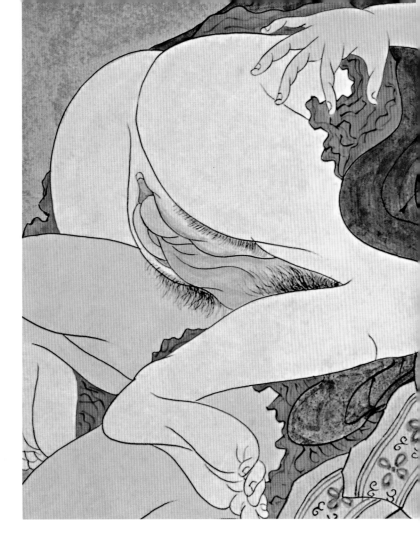

A TYPICAL FRAGMENT OF THE EROTIC LITERARY EXCHANGE WHICH SOME
GEISHA AND MOST OIRAN HAD WITH THEIR PROTECTORS. THIS PIECE IS
MORE POETIC THAN MANY WHILE BEING FIERCELY EROTIC.

How heavy the rain today. How heavy my heart. I am
breaking things and at night my body is on fire. I will call for
the moxa* doctor. Shall I dare write this? What if the
merchant saw these words?

Taking advantage of his position, and mine, the doctor opened his

The maiko is then taken to all her onesan's banquets, introduced to the mistresses of all the teahouses, and to customers and patrons. Once she has received many engagements, she is ready to become a geiko.

Kimono Style

Geisha wear kimono every day as a matter of course—the only social group to do so.

A geisha's kimono constitutes a large part of her art. The presentation of herself in an aesthetic fashion is as important a part of her profession as her singing, her dancing or her musicianship.

Kimono are the single greatest expense in a geisha's budget and about 1 million yen ($10,000) are needed to purchase a minimum wardrobe. A popular geisha changes once or twice during a dinner, and to see her through the change of seasons, she will need about a dozen kimono, along with their coordinated obi.

Motifs have seasonal significance, such as flowers, birds, and insects. And colors too. All Japanese artists are aware of the traditions, and connoisseurs of kimono design appreciate these expressions. Kimono in the spring have a deep crimson lining revealed in the sleeves and at the back of the collar, where it falls away from the neck. The summer brings cooler materials with appropriate colors and patterns. When fall comes the crimson lining is once more seen, as are new designs. A kimono with long sleeves, or one worn to trail behind, will take up to 26 yards of material, 14 inches wide.

The complexity of the obi—the wide sash worn with the kimono—can indicate the social status of the wearer. The position in which it is worn is another clue, and here we see how on a young maiko (right) it is wider and worn high to cover the breasts, and on an older geiko it is more narrow and lower.

The obi is a wide heavy sash that completes a kimono outfit. In a variety of widths and knots, obi reflect the social position of the wearer, as well as fashion trends. For example, obi are tied in front by geisha, in the back by maiko, or apprentices. It is not uncommon for the obi to cost several times more than the kimono itself, and all geisha pride themselves on the quality of this particular article of dress. Hand-woven obi of the highest quality can cost 5 million yen ($50,000).

To help the geisha dress in her elaborate kimono, a dresser (woman or man) comes to the okiya every day. They start by tucking a silk slip around the bare hips, called a *koshimaki*, "hip wrap." Geisha do not wear underwear because a kimono is fairly tight and a line would otherwise show. Instead, the most intimate layer is the traditional koshimaki. Next comes a short-sleeved undershirt, tied shut at the waist, followed by a colored under-robe, coordinated with the kimono; this can be seen when she lifts the hem of her kimono to dance. The under-robe collar must show also. Apprentice geisha wear a red collar, and geisha wear a white one. Finally, the principal job of the dresser is tying the obi. Today, those Japanese wives that wear kimono tie them just below the breasts. Young girls and virgins tie obi highest of all, giving no clue that they even have breasts at all! Geisha tie their obi relatively low, as can be seen on the voluptuous beauties in Utamaro's woodblock prints, with soft, low sashes. Kimono also have to fit the occasion. Maiko and geiko kimono are always made of silk. But at home the informal *yukata*, light cotton kimono, is worn. The geisha's official and smartest outfit of all is the *desho*, a most resplendent trailing black robe made of dyed silk marked by five family crests, with a pattern dyed and embroidered at the hem.

JOY

Visitor this evening
We run up the long corridor
Clicking of clogs.

Only one man,
Only one person to be loved.

I go back to my room,
Retreat, honor,
Lacquered pillow,
Silence.

I hear the watchman's rattle,
Laughter in the next room.

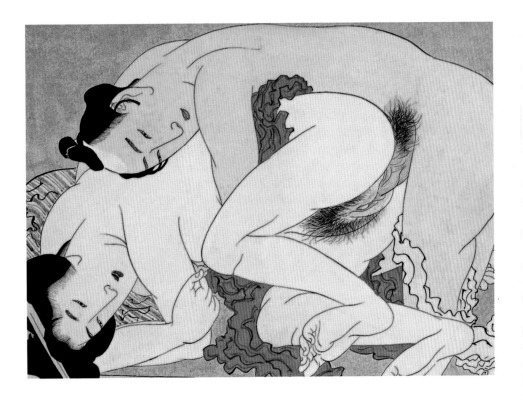

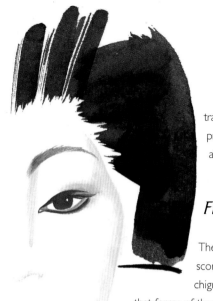

Most Japanese women today, however, never wear traditional dress at all. It is geisha alone who continue to preserve the kimono as the prerogative of a smart woman about town.

Final Touches

The history of Japanese women's hairstyles is complicated: scores of methods of arranging the hair and tying the chignon were constantly devised. A few became so popular that forms of them remain even today, when women have ceased wearing long hair. One style called the *shimada* has been used by geisha for more than a century and a half.

In the mid-'60s, geisha changed to wigs, *katsura*. There were two reasons: a lack of specialized hairdressers, and because geisha change hairstyle with every different kind of dance. Geisha must have at least three different katsura. Each is custom-made from human hair, and costs about half a million yen ($5,000).

Three or four versions of the shimada remain in use today: the "high" shimada, never used by married women, and only by the younger geisha; the "flattened down" shimada, popular chiefly among the older women in the hanamachi; and the "split peach" shimada, or *momoware*, principally worn by maiko during the initial period of training. But once they become geiko, they use the high shimada wig.

The split peach hairstyle is so called because the hair is swept up on top of the head into a large knot which resembles the fruit as if cut in two. Added to the back of the chignon is a piece of fabric, which is left visible in the split. It is always red silk for apprentices, and the sight of it inside the cleft is considered most provocative.

Because the hairdresser takes about forty minutes to prepare the maiko's hair and is very expensive, she visits the salon only once a week.

Once she has made her debut, the new geiko applies her elaborate makeup herself. This can take some time as the white paste must first be mixed with water, and then mirrors arranged so that she can see her back.

To preserve the hairstyle intact, the maiko sleeps on an *omaku*, a black-lacquered wooden pillow, topped by a cushion.

Ornamental hairpins, *kanzashi*, change and are decorated according to the month. They have two pointed pins and decorations are attached. Kanzashi were intended for self-protection: maiko, and geiko, could strike with the pin if they were in danger!

Maiko always wear white makeup but geiko never do, except when they wear a katsura. The white face comes from China, transmitted to ladies of the Japanese Court. Cruse, or white lead, is known to have been used by Chinese women, plus face powder and rouge. During the sixteenth century, pigment was used as a cosmetic by all classes in Japan, and among actors. It gave flatness and an almost mask-like quality. White lead, now known to be toxic, was long ago replaced with modern cosmetic products.

At the maiko debut omisedashi ceremony, a makeup artist will apply the white makeup. Wax is rubbed into the skin of the face, and afterwards into the neck and chest so that the white makeup will adhere. A pale yellow face cream made from nightingale droppings was used in the 1920s. It was believed to be very good for the skin, but was very expensive.

The maiko's face and neck are painted white down from the hairline to her back, and then with a brush from the neck to the breasts and from the nape to the back. Three lines are left unpainted at the back of her neck. This special erotic design, called *sanbon-ashi*, is the reason why geisha wear the collars of their kimono so low in the back. It seems as if the bare skin can just be seen through bars and, according to experts, this makes men much more aware of it.

Eyebrows and eyelids are pencilled in red. Crystallized

A geisha wears the high shimada wig showing an ornamental hair pin, kanzashi, also useful for self-defense. The two lines of white makeup that run from her hairline to her back tantalizingly reveal bare skin as if through bars.

A GEISHA'S SEXUAL SKILLS—ALTHOUGH GENERALLY ENJOYED BY ONE
MAN RATHER THAN MANY, AS WITH THE OIRAN*—WERE DEVELOPED WITH
THE SAME CARE AND ATTENTION TO DETAIL AS MUSIC, POETRY, DIPLOMACY
AND ALL HER OTHER TRADITIONAL SKILLS. THIS SEEMS TO BE AN
INSTRUCTIONAL PIECE, WRITTEN BY AN "OLDER SISTER" OR TUTOR FOR
A NOVICE.

Remember little one, we are more like the things of the sea
but a man is different. You know the old story of the
drawing of a mushroom?* "The more I rubbed it, the bigger
it became. Well then, it wasn't a mushroom was it?" The
scent of a man is like a mushroom, be prepared for that. If he is soft, take
him in your mouth and suck as a calf sucks its mother. Search below with
the tips of your fingers, chase the plums in their sack. Only when he is
hard and angry, the skin taut like a bow string and the purple head
straining like a fish out of water, can you begin.

Slowly, as if it is a delicious thing to you, take the head in your mouth.
Search out the sweet tears of honey with your tongue and as you slide
him deep in your mouth look up and meet his gaze. Oh yes, he will be
watching. Forget the delicacy of the table, suck him noisily. Move up and
down the jade flute* with an insistent rhythm, fingering the shaft if he likes
that. Watch him, meet his gaze, you are the musician in the performance:
see what gives pleasure to your audience. To rest your mouth remove the
instrument from time to time, admiring it with longing eyes. And resume
each time more urgently until you sense the end is near. Oh you will soon
learn that, and then? You are the musician. Sometimes suck him deep
within, the fire juice spurting unseen; another time extend your crimson
tongue between pearly teeth and let the salty waves break across the
pebbles of your tongue. Oh yes, swallow the ocean spume or the balance
(of nature) is disturbed. Why you are moist little one. A tribute to your
teacher I think!

*Oiran were the
courtesans of pre-industrial
Japan. Their training was similar
to that received by geisha, and
included a long apprenticeship
in traditional arts and skills. Like
geisha, highly-educated oiran
often wielded enormous power
and influence, a world away
from the jororu or
humble prostitute.

*The Japanese word for
mushroom, matsuke, is commonly
used for the penis.

*Jade flute is the charming
metaphor for fellatio in
the Chinese and Japanese
erotic traditions.

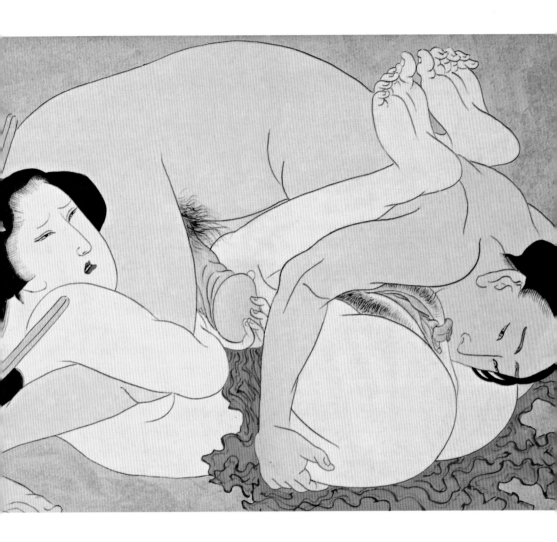

sugar is added to lipsticks for extra shine, and lips are colored to represent a small mouth—considered to be the ideal of feminine beauty.

Maiko and young geiko always wear the long trailed kimono with katsura, white makeup and wooden clogs when they attend the banquets. They would be the laughing-stock of the whole hanamachi if they were improperly dressed.

Hakimono, or footwear, varies according to the occasion. Maiko wear wooden clogs called *okobo*, and *geta*, which are also wooden but not as high as okobo. Apprentice geisha of Kyoto wear a special clog of their own, *koppori*, several inches high and made of black lacquered or plain wood. Being hollow it is quite light in spite of its appearance, and there is usually a small bell fixed inside to tinkle as the wearer trips along. Both maiko and geisha wear *zori*, sandals made of patent leather, with yukata kimono.

Tabi are socks worn with a kimono by both maiko and geiko. Made of white cotton, the big toe of the sock is separated so that sandals or clogs can be worn easily. They are usually made to order to fit their owner, and are designed to retain this shape both on and off the foot.

Footwear too distinguishes maiko (right), with high wooden clogs, from geiko (left). These clogs make quite a sight lined up outside a busy okiya. Note also the one-toed white cotton socks.

The Complete Performance

When ozashiki, or banquets, are held at an ochaya, geisha are requested to attend as professional entertainers. They never eat at a banquet; they only serve, or accept, drinks. During dinner, they dance, sing and play shamisen music, or recite traditional ballads. Conversations are held on equal terms with guests, whatever their position.

Highly trained in hanamachi schools, maiko and geisha
are accomplished in playing most musical instruments,
including the small hand drum, *kotsuzumi*, the Japanese
flute, *fue*, and the best-known Japanese three-stringed
instrument, the *shamisen*. They are also proficient at
traditional dancing, *odori*, with accessories such as the fan
or the parasol, narrative and recitative song and No
theater. (The first female school in Japan was established
in Kyoto in 1871.)

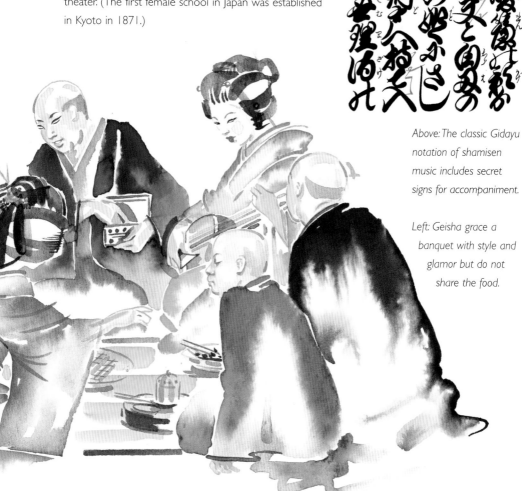

*Above: The classic Gidayu
notation of shamisen
music includes secret
signs for accompaniment.*

*Left: Geisha grace a
banquet with style and
glamor but do not
share the food.*

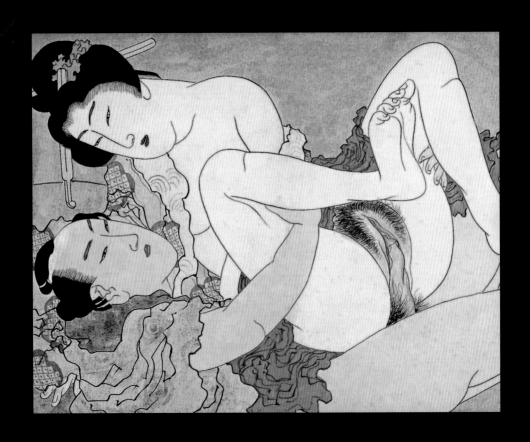

BLACKNESS

The night is black
And I am excited about you.
My love climbs in me, and you ask
That I should climb to the higher room.
Things are hidden in a black night.
Even the dream is black
On the black-lacquered pillow
Even our talk is hidden.

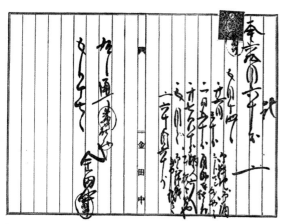

A fascinating teahouse receipt from the 1920s itemizing food, sake, and tips for geisha—described as sake-servers—and their attendants, all totalling 54.10 yen. The tips equaled the cost of the food and drink.

Opening doors, addressing her elders, and entering or leaving a room are all considered part of a geisha's performance, as are *shodo*, a kind of calligraphic art; *kado*, flower arrangement (although generally done by maids); and of course *sado*, the tea ceremony, which dates back to the Heian period and was imported from China. Its objective is not so much to enjoy drinking tea but to display manners and etiquette.

Geisha give public artistic performances, unlike those in the teahouses, in the theaters of the hanamachi. These are spectacular presentations to celebrate special occasions. Dance seasons are mainly in spring and fall, with four performances a day and a tea ceremony is conducted by maiko and geisha before each performance.

The Cherry Dance, *Miyako Odori*, is the best-known popular annual event and takes place in Kyoto during April. The repertoire includes extracts from kabuki plays or is related to kabuki style of theater. Some are based on the traditional Japanese puppet-shows, *bunraku*.

Real money for a geisha comes from having a *danna*, a geisha's financial patron. Once almost all geiko had a danna, but today only about one in five enjoys this security: since World War II, few men are rich enough to be a danna.

Most danna are businessmen or company owners. Her okasan negotiates an agreement in the name of the geisha and the danna pays her a monthly allowance to cover rent and living expenses and also perhaps her kimono. But he also has to pay for her time if he asks her to attend a banquet.

Mizu-age, a euphemism for a maiko's defloration, is a danna's function, or the task is entrusted by the okasan to a man who will treat the young inexperienced girl considerately. Men have been known to pay enormous sums for a mizu-age, especially if they compete and bid for the same girl. In this case, there is no relationship thereafter.

In the modern geisha world, however, the apprentice's deflowering "ceremony" is no longer praticed as such. Sexual relationships are more often than not a matter for maiko and geisha alone. And young geisha seldom obtain a patron until they are in their 20s.

A geisha virtually never has more than one patron. She cannot marry if she is to remain in the profession. Even if she has a danna she is still legally single, and any child by him is considered illegitimate: a danna is usually a man with a respected and powerful position, and will not want his patronage to be public.

The tea ceremony became established as a performance more to express art, culture, and manners, than to drink tea. Greeting guests, making, pouring, and offering the tea are all part of a carefully orchestrated ritual carried out by geisha.

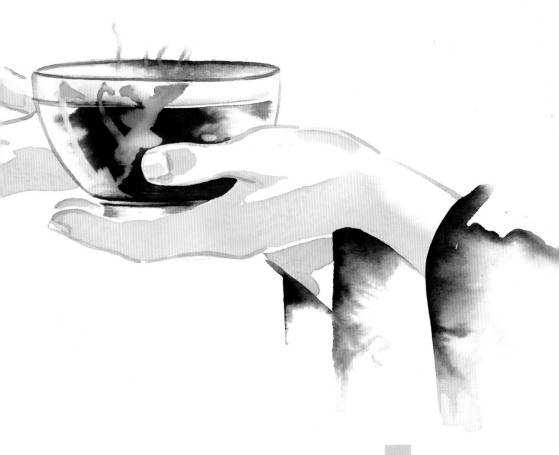

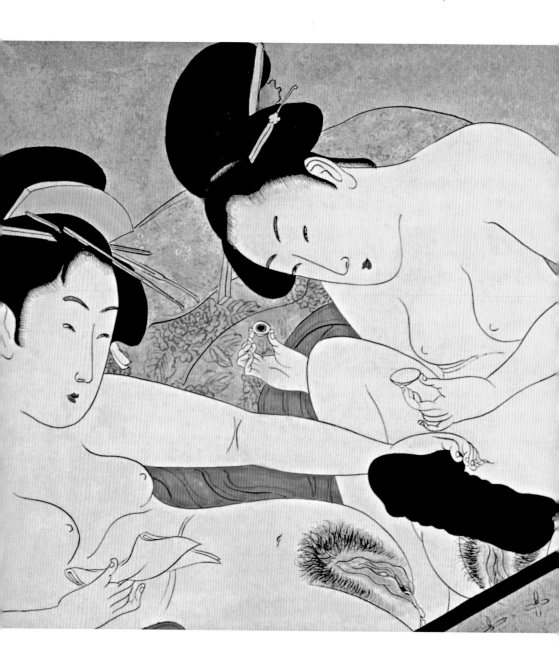

This confessional piece from the nineteenth century could be a diary entry but is more likely to be an erotic literary confection of the kind both geisha and oiran were expected to produce for their protectors. Same sex relationships were common during the long periods of separation endured by many geisha. Little or no guilt was attached to these liaisons, but the universal male interest in girls with girls, and the fact that men find the idea exciting, was well understood in the *ukiyo* or "Floating World."*

*Yoshiwara, or "Floating World," was the pleasure district of Edo which would become modern Tokyo.

*Japanese metaphors are sometimes difficult to translate; "eel" more pleasing than the closer equivalent "leech."

*Dried fish is a common metaphor for the sexually frustrated.

*Harigata were artificial penises, usually made of leather, although there were variants made from buffalo horn or rubber.

She lied of course. There had been no alarm, no fire. I heard the watchman pass as usual. And now the one who is known as eel* is in my room. She is well known in the South-East for preferring women to men and we both know why she has come. Am I not "dried fish,"* longing for love and tired of my own hand? She can have her pleasure of me, it is a journey I have decided to take. Who knows where morning will find me?

She begins so gently. She purrs compliments as she uncovers me. "How white your breasts, how sweet these fruits." Then she sucks at me and I open like a flower. She knows this, and I feel her kisses like butterflies on my thighs. The room is filled with my perfume, the bed damp with my longing. Slowly her kisses come nearer and higher. At last. I give a little cry as she reaches the place, at last. I give myself entirely to passion, pushing up to meet the eel searching among the reeds. Her tongue laps at me, searching every crevice, always returning to polish the little pebble of my longing. I am drenched, all open to her. Very soon now I feel a finger enter love's lower temple, and it is finished. Wave after wave of joy break over me.

I could not say how long I slept. She told me I had been very noisy. I kissed her and noticed a harigata* in her hand. I took it eagerly. Who knows where this journey will end?

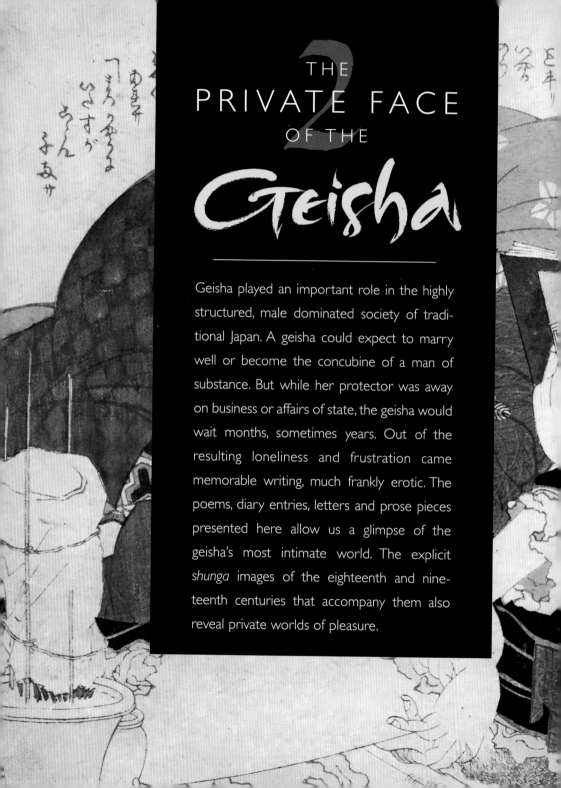

THE
PRIVATE FACE
2 OF THE
Geisha

Geisha played an important role in the highly structured, male dominated society of traditional Japan. A geisha could expect to marry well or become the concubine of a man of substance. But while her protector was away on business or affairs of state, the geisha would wait months, sometimes years. Out of the resulting loneliness and frustration came memorable writing, much frankly erotic. The poems, diary entries, letters and prose pieces presented here allow us a glimpse of the geisha's most intimate world. The explicit *shunga* images of the eighteenth and nineteenth centuries that accompany them also reveal private worlds of pleasure.

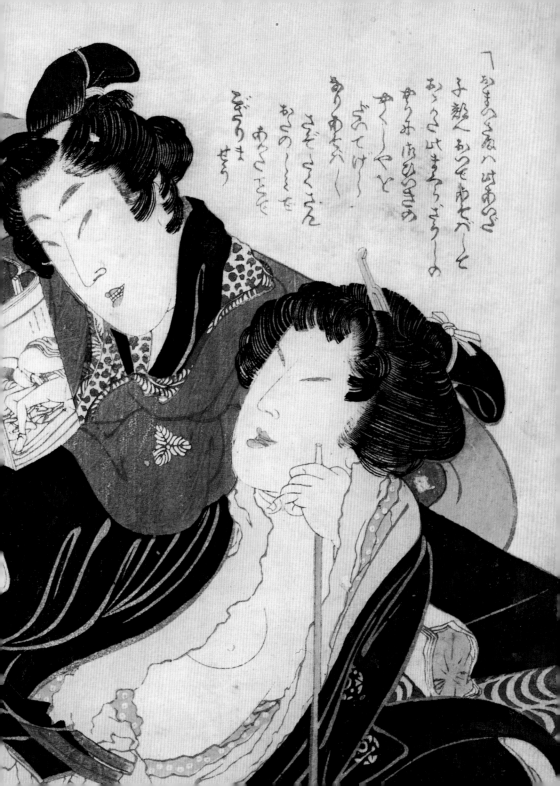

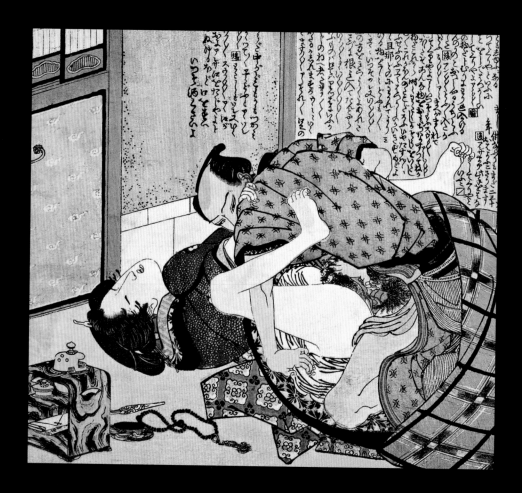

BEFORE MY BIRDS
Geisha song*

I moan for love
Before my birds.
They are also in a cage.

My small complaints
Are sorry like mouse cries.
The birds hop forward to tease me
And I like it
Being so shut in.

The sake is cold
Because my torment
Makes me inefficient.
There is such a thing as grief,
Such a thing as
Being shut in.

*Geisha songs were written to be accompanied by
the shamisen, a three-stringed musical
instrument similar to the lute.

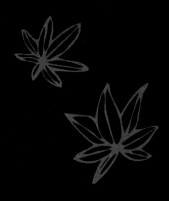

NIGHTINGALE TO PLUM TREE

How the Nightingales sing to the plum trees
And the frogs splash in the water.
That is love.
The call of people and of things
Is everywhere.

Dark Clouds,
Fishing boats,
At the will of the tide,
At the will of the wind.

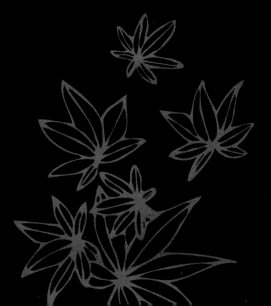

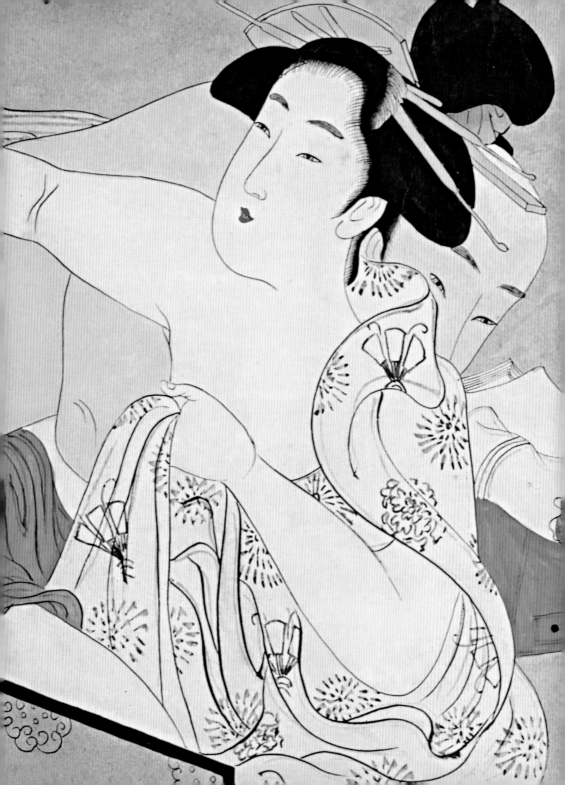

A DELICATELY-WRITTEN PIECE ON THE FAMILIAR SUBJECT OF PARTING.
DREAMS AND THEIR CORRECT INTERPRETATION WERE CONSIDERED TO BE
OF GREAT IMPORTANCE IN PRE-INDUSTRIAL JAPAN. THIS GEISHA MAKES
GENTLE FUN OF THE RATHER OBVIOUS SYMBOLISM IN HER EROTIC DREAM.

H is boat disappears finally behind the island and my longing reaches out across the waves. He left just before dawn as always, an auspicious time, but how cruel life is. How long must I wait for his footfall and his smiling face, to hear his dear voice and to feel the thrill of his caress? I had a dream during the last few hours we slept together. An old servant, one I had not seen since childhood, came with the stick she had used to make the rice gruel and prodded my loins with the damp, round end. It is an old tradition said to make young girls fruitful: I was not surprised at first and laughed. But the servant pushed again until I could feel the hard, sticky tip in the dark hair which protects the shrine of love. Again she pressed, and my lips parted. Now she became more urgent, pressing the churning stick into me deeper each time until I was filled completely. "Stop! What are you doing?" I cried. But the servant answered with his voice, and when I opened my eyes it was his dear face, and his sweet breath, and his lips at my neck. And of the churning stick? I need not say, I think. Nor, lest I blush, will I say more of the hot gruel that soon filled me and hung thick and white about the dark hair and crimson lips. How long my love until I taste that gruel again and hold you in my arms and smell the sweet scent of your body? For now I will make mu tea* and weep.

*Mu tea was made from the flower heads of two special peonies. For this geisha to be drinking it suggests she may be pregnant.

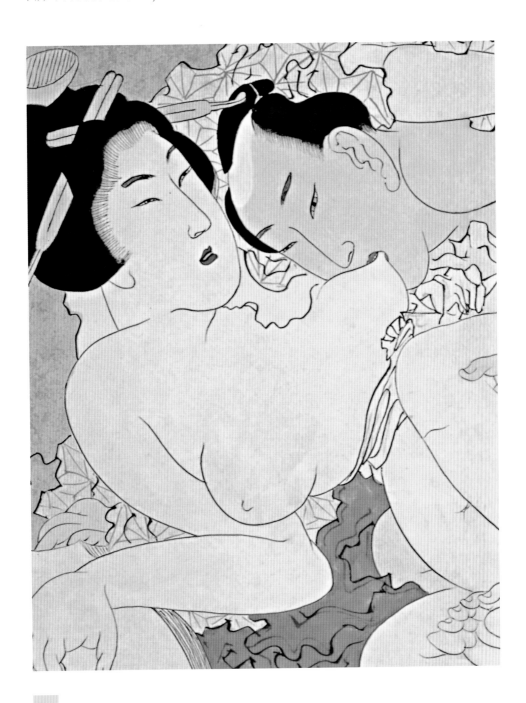

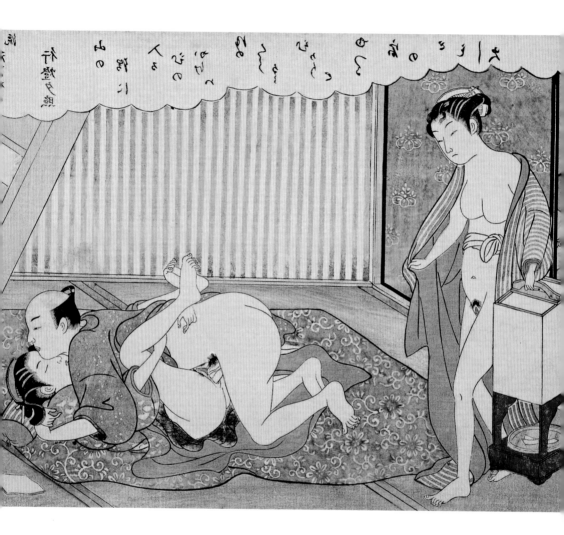

THE WOODEN CONSTRUCTION OF TRADITIONAL JAPANESE BUILDINGS, AND THE EXTENSIVE USE OF PAPER SCREENS TO SEPARATE ROOMS, MEANT THAT ABSOLUTE PRIVACY WAS RARE. AS A RESULT, A WHOLE CULTURE OF VOYEURISM EVOLVED. IN ART, IN LITERATURE—AND IN REALITY—THE INTIMACIES OF LOVERS WERE OFTEN OVERLOOKED OR OVERHEARD BY OTHERS. IN A CULTURE WHICH PLACED SO MUCH IMPORTANCE ON SEX, THIS HAD SOME POSITIVE ADVANTAGES. TRAINEE GEISHA AND *OIRAN* HAD NUMEROUS OPPORTUNITIES TO PERFECT THEIR OWN SEXUAL TECHNIQUE BY OBSERVING AT CLOSE HAND THE BEHAVIOR OF OTHERS.

The old one motioned me to be silent and to sit. She then showed me how to lift the paper flap of the spy hole, and went away chuckling. The merchant from Edo was nearly naked on the *tatami* and so close to me I could smell the sake on his breath. I had never seen Songbird completely naked. Her body was as perfect as her face. She stood smiling before the merchant, caressing the dark little swollen fruits at the point of each breast. Her little tuft of black, silken hair drew my eyes down. Soon her hands were there, stroking the tuft and delicately parting her *bobo kai.** The merchant leaned forward, and with his tongue searched for the pearl within the shell. Suddenly the scene changed. He pulled Songbird down onto the tatami and I saw his plum stalk for the first time, a glistening purple fruit on a dark branch. Songbird tried to taste the plum, but it was too big for her tiny lips. The stranger pushed her down and holding his instrument as if to choke it, rubbed the spade head in the crimson furrow that was open and eager to receive it. The sound this made, like the sucking of waves in rockpools, excited them both to something like fury. She turned round offering herself to him like a mare in season. Nor was her rider slow in mounting her. At first his kimono hid them, but when it slipped away I could see the dark stick garlanded with foam thrusting between her white buttocks. The sound they made—like the wet slapping of a churn—the scent of them like sea and stable—were too much for my senses. It was just as the old one said. I rubbed myself with both hands and at the end my sighs mingled with theirs.

*This means shell, a popular metaphor for the vulva in Japan.

SOUTH-EAST QUARTER

Light affairs become frivolous
At Fukagawa,
My body is frivolous.

A thin uncolored chord on the shamisen.

In intimate Nakatcho Street
Affairs are private,
And the news of our love
Spreads gallantly,
The way of the South-East.
Two lovers are in the little room
And the screen has double hinges.

We pretend worldly fidelity,
Painting moles on each other.

Perhaps
We shall know in heaven.